Contents

☑ KU-757-275

NOTHING CAN
DIM THE LIGHT
THAT SHINES
FROM WITHIN.

MAYA ANGELOU

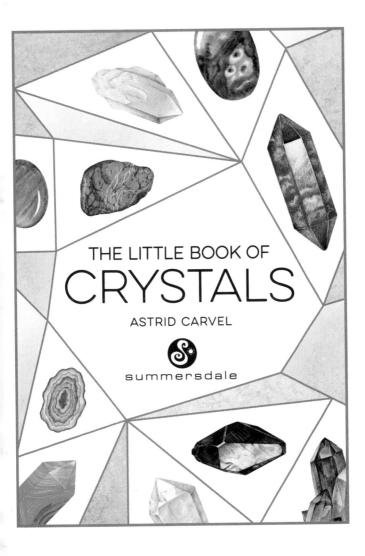

THE LITTLE BOOK OF
CRYSTALS

ASTRID CARVEL

summersdale

THE LITTLE BOOK OF CRYSTALS

An Hachette UK Company
www.hachette.co.uk

Summersdale Publishers Ltd
Part of Octopus Publishing Group Limited
Carmelite House
50 Victoria Embankment
LONDON
EC4Y 0DZ
UK

www.summersdale.com

Printed and bound in Poland

ISBN: 978-1-78685-959-4

Substantial discounts on bulk quantities of Summersdale books are available to corporations, professional associations and other organisations. For details contact general enquiries: telephone: +44 (0) 1243 771107 or email: enquiries@summersdale.com.

INTRODUCTION

Crystals have a mystical, eternal quality and have long been treasured for their beauty. They can refract light, and often have both a translucency and opacity. For thousands of years, they have been prized for their physical and spiritual healing properties. In almost every culture and civilization around the world, crystals of all shapes, colours and sizes have been used in religious rituals, as ornamentation or as talismans of good fortune. Small wonder then that today many of us seem so drawn to these precious and mysterious stones; our fascination with crystals is part of a vast and extensive legacy.

Scratch away the surface and the science behind crystals speaks volumes. All natural crystals vibrate with energy, and for this reason they are used in engineering, from lasers to watches. When these vibrations are used for healing, they have the effect of balancing the energies in the body, allowing for physical, mental or emotional healing. Chinese holistic therapies, in which crystals are integral, describe a system of seven chakras, or energy centres, which are located at the crown of the head, the brow (third eye), throat, heart, stomach (solar plexus), the lower abdomen (or sacral chakra) and the base of the spine (root). By pairing crystals to these chakra points, energies in the body can be unblocked, which not only benefits your general well-being but also alleviates physical ailments.

This guide explains the unique properties of over 40 of the most common crystals and how to experience their healing benefits, from helping with general aches and pains to more specific things, such as finding your inner voice or improving sleep quality.

WHY ARE CRYSTALS SO POPULAR IN THE TWENTY-FIRST CENTURY?

Crystals have always been sought-after objects but they seem more prevalent nowadays, thanks to the rise in popularity of various spiritual and healing practices, including modern white witchcraft.

Many millennials and generation Zs – who perhaps have lost interest in traditional faiths but want to follow a spiritual and metaphysical path that touches upon multiple faiths and ancient practices – are choosing shamanism and crystal healing for a restorative experience to help them deal with the stresses of modern life. You can now purchase a rose quartz heart to help heal heartbreak, a crystal-infused face oil to spritz away stress and crystal wands to safely disperse harmful emissions from your electrical gadgets, for example.

The indefinable magical energy that crystals contain has given them an almost mystical status. While some sceptics believe that they have a placebo effect, it's hard to ignore the factual evidence about the energy that they contain (see pages 16–7).

One of the best things about crystals is that they are easy to come by. You will find a shop selling them in almost every town nowadays, and they are affordable (nothing more than a few pounds or dollars for a small piece of rose quartz or tiger's eye, for example), which means you can build a collection of healing stones for very little outlay. They are also beautiful objects to have around the house, as they catch the light and bring extra sparkle and calming energies to any room.

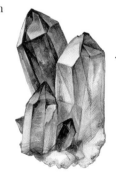

A TIMELINE OF CRYSTAL HISTORY

Our fascination with crystals goes back thousands of years – here's a snapshot of how we have used and benefitted from them throughout history.

 25,000 years BC – There are amulets and talismans in Britain from the Upper Palaeolithic era, many of which are made with Baltic amber (formed over 45 million years ago from tree resin). The use of this gemstone in both jewellery and charms suggests that it was valued for its beauty as well as protective properties.

 14,000 years BC – Dating back to the Upper Palaeolithic era, jet beads, bracelets and necklaces have been unearthed in burial grounds near Thayngen, Switzerland, and in caves in Belgium. The talismanic properties of the beads made them an appropriate grave offering for the dead in early civilization.

 4500–2000 BC – The first recorded references to the use of crystals were likely from the

Ancient Sumerians, who are said to have used gemstones in magic formulas. Magical texts took the form of incantations and describe ritualistic practices performed by these ancient peoples, largely to ward off evil spirits and bad omens in their communities.

3100–330 BC – Ancient Egyptians used crystals, such as lapis lazuli, carnelian, turquoise, clear quartz and emerald, in their amulets and jewellery for health and protection. The dead were buried with a piece of quartz on their forehead to safely guide them to the afterlife, and a necklace of rubies over the heart was intended to bring love into one's life. They also used lapis lazuli and malachite as eye make-up, as shown in their murals and tomb paintings.

1500–1000 BC – In the span of some five hundred years, four sacred Hindu texts were composed, collectively named the "Vedas": *Rig-Veda* (for recitation), *Yajur-Veda* (for liturgy), *Sama-Veda* (for chanting) and *Atharva-Veda* (magic formulas). These texts discuss the use of different crystals to treat certain medical

ailments, as well as their specific properties –
it is said, for example, that emerald will bring
good luck. Ayurvedic medicine is based on
these Vedic texts and is still used today as an
alternative therapy.

800–600 BC – In Ancient Greece, crystals
were used by soldiers and sailors alike to seek
protection from battle and forces of nature. The
Greeks gave names to these crystals, many of
which we still use today; the word "crystal" itself
comes from the Greek word for "ice", as it was
thought that a crystal was simply permanently
frozen water.

315 BC – A text by Theophrastus, titled *Peri
Lithon* (On Stones) was composed, referencing
the healing power of gems and their use in
medical practice.

300 BC – The earliest known written record
of Chinese medicine was composed. Named
the *Huangdi Neijing* (The Yellow Emperor's
Classic of Medicine), it comprised concepts for
traditional Chinese medicine, which remains

the basis of modern practice. Although the system of this medicine is thought to have been around for many thousands of years prior to this, the work outlines a number of important principles for healing practice and refers to energies from the natural world around us. Jade is a particularly important stone in Chinese culture, believed to bring healing and good fortune.

27 BC–AD 476 – Romans used crystals as amulets and talismans to provide them with protection in battle, and attract health and good fortune in their private lives. Crystals were also used in Roman medical treatments.

77 – Pliny wrote *Natural History*, in which he attributed healing values to each crystal.

***c.* 350** – St Epiphanius, Bishop of Salamis in Cyprus, wrote a treatise on the stones mentioned in the Bible. The text, *De Duodecim Lapidibus* (On Twelve Stones), speaks about the 12 stones in the breastplate of the High Priest (Exodus 28) and assigns therapeutic virtues to each one, while also denouncing their supposed "magic powers".

c. **1067–81** – Marbod, Bishop of Rennes, writes his *De Lapidibus* (On Stones), in which he describes 60 gemstones and their magic properties.

1221–84 – Alfonso X, King of Castile and Leon, forms connections between gemstones and astrology in his own lapidary text.

c. **1260** – Saint Albert the Great wrote the treatise *De Mineralibus* (On Minerals) and took a scientific view on their use in healing practices. While focusing heavily on the origin and formation of gemstones, the text also gives weight to their celestial powers.

1300–1600 – During the Renaissance period in Europe, precious and semi-precious stones were used in herbal remedies to heal the sick. The invention of the printing press allowed ancient and contemporary texts on crystals to reach a wider audience than ever. The increased fascination with ancient Greek and Roman cultures fostered a renewed interest in the healing properties of gemstones, as well as their use in sculpture, art and architecture.

c. 1546 – Georg Bauer wrote *De Natura Fossilium*, the first scientific text on minerology, describing the physical characteristics of stones.

1659 – *Gemmarius Fidelius* (The Faithful Lapidary) by Thomas Nicols is published. It argues that gems do not possess any special healing properties. Thus, in the Age of Enlightenment, the use of precious stones for healing and protection fell out of favour in Europe.

Mid-1800s – Investigations into crystal and faith healers and their practices begin to increase scepticism around crystal healing.

1880 – The Curie brothers record the piezoelectric effect (whereby a mechanical force applied to the crystal produces an electrical charge) in quartz.

1921 – Walter Guyton Cady patented the first quartz crystal oscillator, which is widely used in radios, radars and other technologies.

1970s – The advent of New Age culture enjoys a revival of crystals and gemstones for healing practices, which had been side-lined for some time against growing scepticism. Books start to repopularize the use of crystals for spiritual well-being.

Today, our use of crystals continues the long – though by no means exhaustive – history presented here. Crystals are once again becoming part of more mainstream complementary therapies, in addition to their technological uses, and are widely acknowledged for their benefits to our spiritual well-being.

Not only do crystals have a history, but they are history – formed over millions of years and acting as a genuine, physical connection to Earth and the universe that surrounds us.

TO SHINE YOUR BRIGHTEST LIGHT IS TO BE WHO YOU TRULY ARE.

ROY T. BENNETT

HOW CRYSTALS WORK

It can seem like a stretch of the imagination to believe that a humble crystal has the ability to transform your energy levels, help you to find love or heal ills. Crystals are naturally occurring, and they contain piezoelectric and pyroelectric properties that cause them to vibrate. They are also conductors of heat and electricity. It is this innate and perpetual energy that has led to crystals being used for centuries for medicinal purposes, as recorded in the Bible and Chinese medical texts.

We all emit vibrations – high when we're stressed or low when we're feeling sad. Crystals have the effect of balancing the vibrations in the body or in the environment and encourage a renewed sense of calm and well-being. They also help to restore the body's natural healing mechanisms. This type of non-invasive healing is called vibrational medicine. Crystals are often selected according to their properties and colour, and applied to a chakra point on the body. These chakra points are located as follows.

Chakra	Location	Colour	Emotional and physical associations
Root	Base of spine	Red	Feeling grounded, independent
Sacral	Just below navel	Orange	Acceptance, well-being, pleasure
Solar plexus	Base of ribcage	Yellow	Confidence, self-control, self-esteem
Heart	Centre of chest	Green	Love, joy and inner peace
Throat	Base of throat	Blue	Communication, self-expression
Third eye	Above and between brows	Indigo	Intuition, decision-making
Crown	Top of head	Violet	A feeling of connection, spirituality

THE POWER OF COLOUR

To discern a crystal's health benefits, it is important to study its colours. Using colours for therapeutic purposes, where hues and light are employed to positively affect a person's mood and mental health, has been practised since ancient times. This medical practice is known as chromotherapy. Think about how you feel when you enter a bright yellow room and how it raises your happiness levels, almost giving you a shake to wake you up. Conversely, a pale blue or green space can have an instant calming and soothing effect, like when you look out to sea.

Chromotherapy – the basics

Chromotherapy is a fascinating therapy with its origins dating back to Ancient Egypt and China, and it's still used today as a holistic treatment. Modern-day chromotherapy uses lights to transmit colours to the patient. Each colour is said to benefit our physical and mental well-being in different ways.

- Red stimulates body and mind, and is used to alleviate circulation problems and ease cold symptoms.

- Orange gives an energy boost and has been used in conjunction with other therapies to stimulate the lungs and respiration. It's also used to kindle brain activity and creative expression.

- Yellow is for positivity, helping to dispel negative thoughts and sadness.

- Green is a serene, soothing colour associated with positive mental well-being.

- Blue is calming and soothing for both body and mind, reducing inflammation particularly in areas pertaining to the throat.

- Purple calms the body and mind, aids sleep, and awakens intuition.

COLOUR IS A POWER WHICH DIRECTLY INFLUENCES THE SOUL.

WASSILY KANDINSKY

HOW TO SELECT YOUR CRYSTALS

There is no scientific way to choose crystals but, as with everything in life, try to go with your instincts. Spend time picking them up; see which ones hold your attention. Set an intention with the crystal(s) that you choose. You can do this while meditating and holding the stone in your hand as you state what you need from the crystal's energy.

The myriad different choices available may seem overwhelming at first, but a crystal's colour will give you a clue to its properties. Red is associated with courage, so carry red jasper if you need a bravery boost. Orange aids creativity and yellow instils happiness. Turn to green to balance the emotions. Blue allows clear communication, indigo helps you to tune into your intuition and violet can increase your spiritual awareness.

If you have a specific requirement, however, you can refer to the A–Z of crystals in the following pages to discover the right one for your needs.

HOW TO CLEANSE YOUR CRYSTALS

Some practitioners of crystal healing advocate the importance of cleansing and preparing your crystals before use, so that any negative or old energy is removed, as if giving it a reboot. There are several ways to do this including the following.

Rinse in running water for a minute and leave
to dry in the fresh air – this is not suitable for
brittle stones, as they could erode in the water.

Submerge in salt water for
24 hours and leave to air-dry.

Bathe in moonlight or sunlight for 12 hours.

AN A–Z OF
Essential crystals

Each entry in this A–Z explains how to identify a crystal, where they are sourced, what they are best suited for and how they can be used in healing practices. It also explains the chakra zone that each crystal pertains to (see page 17 for the chakra zones chart).

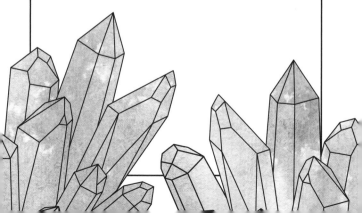

Agate

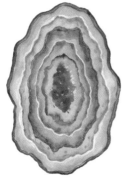

Origin: Sicily

Colour: There are many colours, but the most prevalent are green, pink, brown, blue and black

Birthstone for: June

Chakra zone: Heart

Best for: Stability, protection and emotional security

From the Babylonians to the medieval times – and right up to the present day – agate has been used to protect against bad energy and natural disasters. In Chinese medicine it was traditionally used to clear negative thoughts; nowadays, it is still considered to have powers of protection, as well as the capacity to unblock emotional centres to help release tension in the heart and the throat, thus improving emotional connection and helping you to find your voice – both literally and figuratively.

Also known as silicon dioxide, and part of the chalcedony family, there are many varieties of agate. Its name comes from the river Achates in Sicily, where fragments of it were first discovered among Neolithic remains.

CRYSTAL TIPS

Make an elixir by dropping a piece of agate into a glass of tap water; allow its positive energies to permeate the liquid, before taking out the crystal and drinking the water. The gentle energy that radiates from the crystal will disperse around your body as you drink, invoking a sense of calm and inner peace.

Place pieces of agate around your bedroom to balance emotional and sexual energy.

Wear an agate pendant as a protective talisman for potentially difficult or emotionally charged situations, such as meeting an ex-partner or taking an exam.

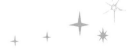

Amber

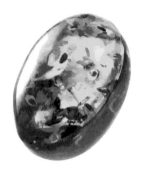

Origin: **Poland, Germany, Russia and the UK**

Colour: **Dark gold**

Birthstone for: **May**

Chakra zone: **Solar plexus**

Best for: **Concentration, purification and health**

Amber has the translucent quality of crystal, but it is actually fossilized resin from pine trees. This stone has historically been used as protection against negative forces or seen as a good-luck talisman to ancient peoples.

In more recent years, it has been prized for the exceptional energies it discharges when under friction. Amber has been shown to be beneficial in relieving anxiety, uplifting negative moods, and even in removing pain and inflammation when placed against the skin; for this reason, the stone remains popular in alternative medicinal practice.

CRYSTAL TIPS

Burn amber incense during an evening meditation or a gentle yoga session, as the aroma will soothe and relax the mind and body, and encourage a restful night's sleep.

- -

A piece of amber held against the skin is said to release succinic acid, an antioxidant, which is believed to slow the effects of ageing by boosting the body's lipids to promote elasticity.

- -

Use this stone in teething necklaces to ease pain and irritability – as well as reduce saliva production by stimulating the thyroid gland – and soothe the inflammation of the mouth and cheeks during this stage in a baby's development.*

Always check with a health practitioner as to the latest safety guidelines on the use of amber teething necklaces.

Amethyst

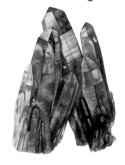

Origin: Worldwide

Colour: Purple

Birthstone for: February

Chakra zone: Third eye and crown

Best for: Trust, intuition and spirituality

With its rich history and signature deep-purple hue, amethysts have been held in high esteem for many centuries. Historically, they were treasured by the Neolithic people in Europe as a decorative emblem, while the Ancient Greeks and the Romans used amethysts in their jewellery and amulets. Associated with wealth and luxury, its use has largely been in jewellery, especially in religious and aristocratic circles.

A protective stone, amethyst helps to purify the mind, and eases stress and anxiety. The crystal also facilitates creativity and communication, so can be used as a talisman for focus and success.

CRYSTAL TIPS

Place amethysts in a living space, like a family room, to assist in familial bonding activities, and provide a feeling of confidence and calm, necessary for open communication.

Keep a piece of amethyst in an office space to bring intuition when making difficult decisions in business and to act as stress relief in challenging environments.

Place amethysts in the bathroom – or next to you, on the side, while having a bath – to alleviate anxiety and help to stimulate feelings of relaxation.

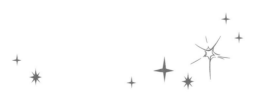

Aquamarine

(from the beryl family, see page 34)

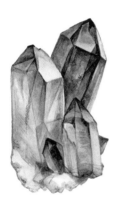

Origin: **Brazil, Russia, Kenya, Madagascar and the Midwestern US**

Colour: **Blue and cyan**

Birthstone for: **March**

Chakra zone: **Throat and heart**

Best for: **Stress relief, soothing and deepening meditative states**

From the Latin *aqua marinus,* or 'sea water', aquamarine was often used by Roman sailors to generate good fortune, fearlessness and protection from the elements. Because of its flowing, peaceful energy, aquamarine is still thought to be effective in moving and purifying your own energy, thus aiding emotional healing and deepening meditative states. Its ability to heal and soothe can also help to relieve stress and protect your energy from being drained by negativity.

CRYSTAL TIPS

Aquamarine is the stone of breath and the lungs, and as a cooling stone can be helpful in soothing respiratory issues. By wearing an aquamarine pendant, the stone can be kept close to its key chakras and act on the affected areas. If suffering from eye irritations, it may be useful to place aquamarine gemstones on the eyelids for 20 minutes each night before bed.

Carry an aquamarine stone around with you in stressful situations to help soothe your nerves and dispel negative energy directed towards you.

Hold an aquamarine stone in one hand while meditating to reach deeper truths. Light turquoise aquamarine, in particular, is known to impart refreshing energy, balance and peace during meditation.

Aventurine

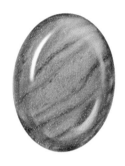

Origin: India

**Colour: Most commonly
green, but also orange,
brown, yellow, blue,
grey, white and red**

Birthstone for: September

Chakra zone: Solar plexus

**Best for: Good
fortune, opportunity
and confidence**

Known in the gemstone world as one of the luckiest stones, the green aventurine is a must-have for inviting good luck and prosperity into your life, and is thought to be more powerful than the other colours. In fact, so powerful are its properties of good fortune that you need only be near a green aventurine to derive its benefits. This stone does not only bring good luck, but also opportunity, stimulating you to release old habits and move forward with confidence to embrace change.

CRYSTAL TIPS

Keep an aventurine gemstone in your pocket so that it is always close and able to transfer its fortune and opportunity in any situation.

Green aventurine is known for its soothing properties, so having it nearby helps to balance the emotional body, as well as calming nervousness, anger and irritation.

Wear a necklace made of blue aventurine beads close to your throat to balance the chakras that help with communication. Alternatively, wear jewellery of white aventurine stones to deepen your spirituality.

Red aventurine is believed to boost sexual desire and vitality when placed near the three lower chakras or the solar plexus.

Beryl

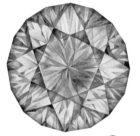

Origin: Parts of Europe, South America, South Africa, the Middle East and the US

Colour: There are many colours, but the most prevalent are green, blue, yellow, pink and clear

Birthstone for: May

Chakra zone: Crown and solar plexus

Best for: Protection, stress relief and spiritual healing

Beryl is clear in its pure form; the many different impurities in the gem give it its varied colouration. Popular colours include pink (morganite), yellow (heliodor), green (emerald) and blue (aquamarine). Red (bixbite) is very rare, having been found in just a few locations.

For many centuries, beryl has been worn as a personal talisman, thought to protect against dark forces and evil spirits. Nowadays, beryl is a gem which helps with day-to-day stresses and emotional baggage. In its various forms, it can relieve a multitude of anxieties and also promote physical healing in the crown, throat and solar plexus.

CRYSTAL TIPS

Though it comes in a variety of forms and colours, all types of beryl are known to ease stress and anxiety. When worn close to the body, for instance in jewellery, beryl is known to stimulate your mind in research or philosophical studies and to confer gentle, calming energies.

Place beryl in the bedroom to enhance intimacy with your partner or in the living room to bring positive, uplifting energy.

The benefits of beryl can also be gained through an elixir: drop into a glass of water for a few minutes to allow the properties of the crystal to disperse in the liquid before removing it and drinking; in this form, the crystal can act as a sedative and open the mind to new information.

Blue lace agate

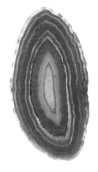

Origin: **Africa**

Colour: **Blue**

Birthstone for: **June**

Chakra zone: **Throat and third eye**

Best for: **Inner stability, composure and maturity**

Historically, blue lace agate was used by the Babylonians for healing amulets and ornamentation, and its medicinal uses extend back to the ancient Greek and Egyptian civilizations. Its natural swirling design reflects the circular, flowing energies it gives out, which calm, uplift and elevate.

It is sometimes called "the earth rainbow" for its concentric bands of blues, whites and even browns.

CRYSTAL TIPS

Keep blue lace agate close at hand when speaking in public, or if intending to share thoughts or ideas with strangers. Known as the "stone of the diplomat", it is believed that this crystal calms the mind and strengthens sensitivities. Its warm, protective properties also encourage security and self-confidence.

Place the crystal on the abdomen – or use as an elixir by putting it in some tap water and removing it before drinking – to stimulate the digestive system and relieve gastritis. Due to its soothing qualities, it can also help to heal skin disorders and itchiness from insect bites.

Place a cold agate in the middle of the forehead to relieve the symptoms of fever or to help guard against sleepwalking.

Carnelian

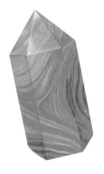

Origin: Brazil, India, Siberia and Germany

Colour: Brownish-red

Birthstone for: August

Chakra zone: Sacral

Best for: Motivation, endurance, leadership and courage

Carnelian is a variety of chalcedony and its colour varies from pale pinkish-orange to a deep rusty brown. Its name is thought to originate from the Latin word for "flesh", though it could also come from the Cornelian cherry, which it closely resembles.

From antiquity to the present day, this stone has been thought to help speakers to become bold and eloquent, transferring courage and physical power to its wearer. However, due to its glowing and vibrant colour, it has also been linked to passion, love and desire.

CRYSTAL TIPS

Wear as jewellery over the heart to stimulate a constant flow of warmth and support when you are in the spotlight.

Place a carnelian in your bath and infuse the water with its healing properties as an effective boost before a big event in your life. To maximize the results of this, try also saying an affirmation to yourself, such as: "I am confident and self-assured."

Use a carnelian during meditative practice by holding it just below the navel when seated. Allow yourself to close your eyes and sit quietly until you feel that you are ready to focus your energy on some of the thoughts in your mind. Let the vibrant energy of the stone bring you confidence when faced with a difficult task.

Chrysoprase

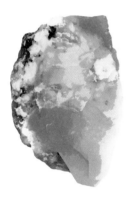

Origin: **Indonesia, Western Australia, Tanzania, Germany, Poland, Russia, Brazil and the US**

Colour: **Green**

Birthstone for: **July**

Chakra zone: **Heart**

Best for: **Optimism, compassion and joy**

Originating from the ancient Greek words *chrys* (gold) and *prase* (green), this stone was historically used to make seals, signets and decorative jewellery, because of its vivid green hue.

These crystals tend to vary widely between each other – from bright "apple" greens to pale-yellowish hues – and are known for promoting happiness, joy and self-acceptance, alongside forgiveness and compassion toward others. The crystal is thought to be particularly effective for easing anxiety and stress, as well as supporting romance and relationships through its connection to the heart chakra.

CRYSTAL TIPS

Place this crystal in the bath for an extra dose of stress relief and relaxation. Hold the stone over your chest while you soak in the water, and contemplate your intentions and goals to encourage positive thinking. This will also help to heal heartbreak and loneliness, due to its connection with the heart chakra.

In meditation, hold a chrysoprase in each hand and visualize positive vibrations flowing through your chakras to create alignment in your body.

Wear this stone or keep it close at hand to maximize its benefits, both in physical healing and positive energies.

Citrine

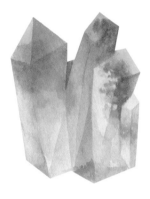

Origin: Brazil, Africa, Madagascar, Spain, Russia, France, Scotland and the US

Colour: Yellow

Birthstone for: November

Chakra zone: Root, sacral and solar plexus

Best for: Joy, creativity and abundance

Derived from the French word for "lemon" *(citron)*, citrine is a bright and sunny yellow crystal which emanates positivity, creativity and light. From the Ancient Romans, who used this as an ornamental gem, to the Art Deco era, when it was popular in jewellery, citrine has maintained its popularity because of its joyous appearance and positive energy.

This crystal is one of abundance and manifestation, attracting prosperity and wealth, and is often referred to as the Merchant's or Success Stone. It is also popular with artists for stimulating creativity and imagination.

CRYSTAL TIPS

Use this stone while meditating to strengthen mental output, and amplify your intellectual acuity and creativity.

Keep a small amount of citrine in your purse or wallet to maximize your prosperity and wealth.

Place citrine in your bedroom to bring light and abundance into the area. Keeping the crystal in a workspace or office can add prosperity and creativity to your workflow. Alternatively, placing the stone in a child's bedroom can offer feelings of security.

Wear this crystal anywhere on your body to see its benefits, though putting it as close as possible to the solar plexus chakra will enhance your creativity.

Clear quartz

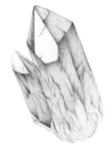

Origin: **Worldwide**

Colour: **Clear**

Birthstone for: **April**

Chakra zone: **Crown**

Best for: **Clarity, focus and visualization**

As one of the most abundant minerals in the world, clear quartz has been treasured across a broad range of cultures and geographies. In many cases, this crystal has been seen to signify purity and space, and has been symbolic of a vessel, carrying spirits and positive forces. Some ancient cultures believed that quartz crystals were alive – even to the point where they would take a breath, albeit once a century.

The transparent nature of this stone reflects the clarity of thought which it offers; it is useful in expanding consciousness, and facilitating clear and open communication. Though it is particularly aligned with the crown chakra, it is known to resonate on some level with all chakras. Clear quartz is used in electrical engineering for its pyroelectric and piezoelectric properties – items such as computer chips, circuit boards and radios all contain quartz.

CRYSTAL TIPS

Set this crystal on your third-eye chakra to establish clarity in your meditation. Try repeating mantras like, "I am clear about my goals and motivations," as this will strengthen the visualization of your objectives and solidify the intentions of your practice.

Hold this crystal in the palm of your hand and focus on what you want to transfer to it. The crystal will take on your intentions and help you to manifest your goals through its amplification. It is, however, important to cleanse the stone regularly (see page 22), in order to retain its positive energy.

Diamond

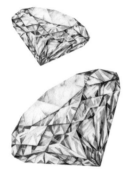

Origin: Primarily Russia, Botswana, the Democratic Republic of Congo (DRC), Australia and Canada

Colour: Clear

Birthstone for: April

Chakra zone: Crown

Best for: Amplification, strength and positivity

From the ancient Greek word *adamas* (unbreakable), diamonds have been admired and venerated throughout history in religious icons and ornate jewellery. As the hardest known naturally occurring substance, diamonds command the powers of strength and fortitude – as well as purity and innocence.

Due to their composition, diamonds are great amplifiers of energy, absorbing thoughts and feelings, and radiating them outward. Remaining positive while holding or wearing diamonds will help to project empowering thoughts to those around you.

CRYSTAL TIPS

Wear or carry a diamond only after some level of introspection, as these precious gems are known to amplify emotions, whether positive or negative. Simply removing the crystal when you are in a negative frame of mind can alleviate its power.

- -

Hold a diamond in your palm while meditating to bring clarity of mind and to amplify your intentions.

- -

Keep a diamond around in warm and congenial environments to infuse the space with feelings of joy, light and openness. Once again, be aware that when negative energies are dominating the space, these may be amplified by this crystal.

Fluorite

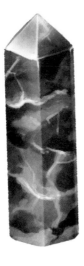

Origin: Worldwide, but largely in South Africa, Mexico, China, Mongolia, Spain and Russia

Colour: Various (commonly green and purple)

Birthstone for: None directly, but related to springtime

Chakra zone: Third eye and heart

Best for: Peacefulness, clarity and calm

Fluorite (See yellow fluorite on page 104) typically contains green and purple colours, each offering different – though synergistic – properties. The green in the crystal cleanses the heart chakra by aligning the heart and mind, while the purple opens and stimulates the third eye chakra, offering a path for spiritual expansion.

This crystal is particularly useful for those who require focus in their life, and operate in stressful and challenging environments, as fluorite promotes a calm and peaceful state of mind.

CRYSTAL TIPS

Place this stone near to you when you are sleeping or meditating to allow for mental clarity and harmony between the chakras. Fluorite will also help to guide you from feelings of anxiety to tranquillity by cleansing your mind and the environment around you. This stone should leave you feeling free from mental blocks, and able to think clearly and creatively.

Wear fluorite in your jewellery to neutralize and absorb negative energy, such as stress and anxiety, and receive a constant flow of positive energy. It is also beneficial to wear this stone alongside other healing crystals, as it is known to magnify their effects.

Garnet

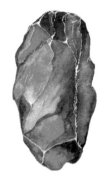

Origin: India, China and the US

Colour: Most commonly, red, orange, brown and pink

Birthstone for: January

Chakra zone: Heart

Best for: Energy, health and well-being

Garnets have been used for personal ornamentation since the Ancient Egyptians. Though it is found across the world in different varieties, the most popular form of the stone is in its luminous red and orange hues.

Garnets are popularly seen as being linked with romance and matters of the heart, because of the intensity of their colour and also its powers of attraction in love. This stone can also be used to find balance, as well as clarity and enlightenment in meditation.

CRYSTAL TIPS

Lie flat on your back on a yoga mat, with your legs outstretched, and place a garnet crystal over the pubic bone, another on the heart and the final one between the feet to feel all seven chakras easing back into alignment. With this new sense of balance, visualize the stones infusing with you in your practice, transferring to you their powerful energy.

Wear a garnet as jewellery to sharpen your perceptions of others and to bestow self-confidence. By keeping the chakras aligned, garnets can also transmute your energy to a beneficial state, and maintain health and well-being.

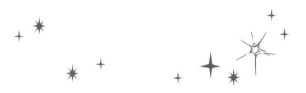

Hematite

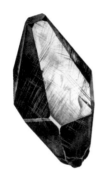

Origin: China, Australia, Brazil, India, Russia, Ukraine, South Africa and the US

Colour: Metallic grey or red

Birthstone for: February and April

Chakra zone: Root

Best for: Grounding, manifestation and focus

The metallic, glimmering surface of this crystal means that it is often associated with moonlight and the stars. Hematite reminds us to stay grounded and to connect with the world around us. Perhaps more important than ever, in our hectic, technological age, this stone can be used to clear away toxicity and keep our feet firmly on the ground.

Hematite is stable and reliable in its positive energies, so it is useful to keep this crystal in your proximity to feel its cool and calm presence at all times.

CRYSTAL TIPS

Clear your meditative space from distractions by putting away your phone, diary and other modern-day gadgets. Light a candle and lie on your back with your legs outstretched. Place a stone on your lower abdomen, and hold one in each hand for maximum grounding effect. Inhale deeply and exhale, repeating a mantra such as, "I am grounded and centred on this earth." The stone will bolster your strength as you are saying this.

Wear this crystal or keep it close by to help manifest your aims and intentions, while drawing away any negative energy and toxicity in your environment.

Iolite

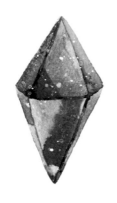

Origin: Australia (Northern Territory), Brazil, Canada, India, Madagascar, Myanmar, Namibia, Sri Lanka, Tanzania and the US

Birthstone for: Associated with winter

Colour: Purple, grey and blue

Chakra zone: Third eye

Best for: Balance, confidence and creativity

Known as the "Stone of the Muses", iolite promotes creativity and self-assurance in actions. It is also known as a "vision stone", as it acts almost as a compass to guide us spiritually and physically in the world. Iolite activates the creative side of the mind and often inspires self-expression through song, movement and the written word.

Iolite provides a sense of balance, as well as a strengthened resolve, so its energies are best delivered in times of uncertainty and disorder.

CRYSTAL TIPS

Place iolite in quiet, calm and meditative spaces to harness the maximum benefit from the crystal. In this environment, the stone will both revitalize and energize the space with peace and harmony, while also supporting you in your endeavours.

Wear iolite in your jewellery to benefit from its effects at all times. The more this stone is worn, the greater the effect on your energies, so it is advisable to wear it as much as possible in times of healing and when you require guidance in your life.

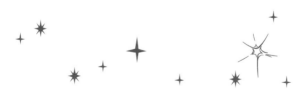

Jade

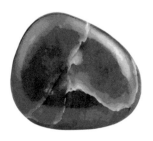

Origin: Myanmar, Guatemala, Mexico and Russia

Colour: Green

Birthstone for: March

Chakra zone: Heart

Best for: Wisdom, success and wealth

Jade is seen as a good-luck charm in the world of crystals, due to its ability to deliver prosperity and abundance. Historically, this stone was highly prized across Mexico, Central and South America, and perhaps most famously China, where it has been used extensively in the country's art and religious iconography. Across time and geographies, this stone has also been used medicinally for kidney and bladder issues. Now the stone signifies peace, wisdom and wealth, and helps to harmonize emotional and physical well-being.

CRYSTAL TIPS

Place jade over your heart chakra while meditating to balance your well-being and to stabilize your emotional responses to those around you. A jade necklace which positions the gem directly at the centre of the breastbone works well for this.

Keep a piece of jade in your pocket or close to you throughout the day, particularly in busy and unfamiliar locations, as the gem offers a form of protection.

Place jade under your pillow while you are sleeping to induce lucid dreams, and to encourage a deep and restful sleep.

Place a piece of jade in your purse or mix it with some coins to attract greater luck, prosperity and abundance.

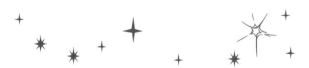

Jasper

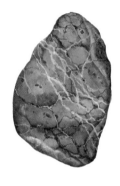

Origin: India, Russia, Kazakhstan, Indonesia, Egypt, Madagascar, Australia, Brazil, Venezuela, Uruguay and the US

Colour: Brown, yellow and red

Chakra zone: Root

Birthstone for: March

Best for: Grounding, cleansing and calm

Since ancient times, jasper has been used by shamans and healers to make protective talismans and amulets; the deep brown and red colours of the stone have been seen as masculine and earthy, connecting the vital lifeblood of the body with the earth beneath us. We still acknowledge this stone as one of the most powerful for connecting with the world around us, and it reminds us to keep our feet on the ground and be appreciative of nature.

CRYSTAL TIPS

Place jasper on the root chakra to stabilize and energize the body. By putting it over each chakra point in turn, the stone is known to cleanse, boost and realign the chakras and the aura, balancing your energies and grounding the body.

Wear jasper in jewellery or carry it close to the body to alleviate stress and induce tranquillity. Its cleansing effect eliminates negative energy and stabilizes the aura. Place jasper under your pillow to reduce nightmares and allow for a more restful sleep. It is also ideal when used as a rubbing stone before bed to soothe nerves and calm the mind.

Jet

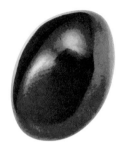

Origin: Russia, India, the UK, Spain, Germany, France, Poland and the US

Colour: Black

Birthstone for: January

Chakra zone: Root and third eye

Best for: Support, protection and harmony

Jet is a powerful and protective stone, from which you can draw strength when you are feeling vulnerable or weak, or facing difficult situations. This stone helps to release feelings of anger, fear and worry in a positive way. Used extensively in the Victorian era in mourning jewellery, the stone is widely known for its ability to heal grief, though perhaps less so for its harmonizing properties and capacity to restore balance in life. The stone has also been used extensively for protection against negative energies; however, it must be regularly cleansed when used for such a purpose.

CRYSTAL TIPS

Wear jet as jewellery or keep a piece nearby through periods of pain and distress to feel its soothing and supportive effects.

Place the stone on the forehead – or a piece of jet on each eye – to treat headaches and migraines. The soothing and cooling effects of the crystal should alleviate pain and ease suffering.

Jet should be frequently cleansed of its negative energy and recharged by placing the stone in sea salt overnight, or by burying it in the ground under the light of a full or new moon.

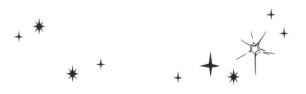

Labradorite

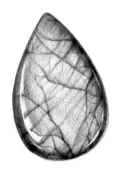

Origin: Canada, Australia, Madagascar, Mexico, Norway, Russia and the US

Colour: Grey-black, with colourful iridescence

Birthstone for: August

Chakra zone: Third eye and crown

Best for: Curiosity, magic and escapism

Named after the place where it was first discovered (Labrador, Canada), this stone was initially popular with missionaries for its particular iridescence. The Inuits too valued the stone for its colour, which led to legends that the Northern Lights had been captured inside it. Seen as a stone of magic, due to its inner mystical light, it is popular with people looking to seek knowledge and guidance in the universe. It is also excellent for awakening further spiritual capabilities.

CRYSTAL TIPS

Hold a piece of labradorite in each hand while you meditate to feel your consciousness expanding and open your mind to the world around you. While performing this meditation, it is advisable to keep a piece of smoky quartz under or between your feet, in order to keep yourself grounded.

Keep a stone in the workplace to bring out the best in those around you and to make your colleagues more congenial. It also allows its holder to curb antisocial tendencies and temper more negative traits.

Wear or carry labradorite to allow any innate spiritual powers to surface and to expand intuitive abilities.

Lapis lazuli

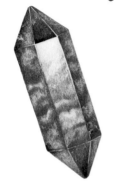

Origin: Afghanistan, Russia, Chile, Italy, Mongolia and the US

Colour: Blue

Birthstone for: September

Chakra zone: Third eye and throat

Best for: Truth, awareness and wisdom

Since ancient times, lapis lazuli has been held in high regard for its rich, royal blue colour and its use as a dye in make-up and clothing. This stone was particularly prized in Ancient Egypt, and used extensively in regal ornamentation and jewellery. With such a rich history, it is not surprising that the stone remains popular today, used widely as a conduit for wisdom, judgement and truth. Lapis lazuli is a powerful crystal for enhancing intellectual activity, and it stimulates the desire for knowledge and learning.

CRYSTAL TIPS

Carry this crystal around with you or wear it as jewellery to attract success, promotion and lasting recognition in your field. Its ability to stimulate and enrich your mind with learning will increase the likelihood of your achievement.

Use this stone in meditative practice to broaden your mind to past-life connections and to act as a catalyst for your spiritual awareness. This stone will help you to access the knowledge of past lives and inspire personal progress.

Keep this stone close in situations where you require calm and loving communication, such as with energetic or distressed young people. This stone will aid honesty and bring harmony to difficult relationships.

Malachite

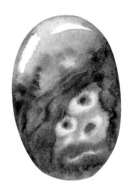

Origin: Russia, Zaire, Australia, South Africa, Germany, Romania, Chile, Mexico and the US

Colour: Green

Birthstone for: Associated with springtime

Chakra zone: Heart and throat

Best for: Protection, balance and transformation

As a stone of protection, malachite is known to absorb negative energies and pollutants from both the body and the atmosphere around it. Perhaps more necessary now than ever before, this stone safeguards against pollutants, noise, harsh lighting and radiation from technological equipment. It also balances the mind in stressful environments, acting as a layer of protection and calm. However, this stone must be used with caution and only in its polished form; it is important not to breathe in its dust, which is hazardous to health.

CRYSTAL TIPS

Hold a polished malachite stone in each hand to aid concentration and to help balance the mind to relieve feelings of confusion. While there, the stone will also help to absorb negativity from the body, and therefore should be cleansed regularly by being left out in the sun for a few hours.

Wear malachite on the body to assist with multitasking and to increase focus on each task individually. The stone should also help to support you in difficult activities at hand. It is worth noting that this rock is soft and easily damaged, so a necklace or earrings are to be preferred to a ring or a bracelet.

Milky quartz

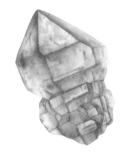

Origin: **Across Europe, Russia and Siberia**

Colour: **White – translucent to opaque**

Birthstone for: **January**

Chakra zone: **Crown**

Best for: **Healing, confidence and relaxation**

Sometimes called the "snow quartz" for its icy-looking appearance, this crystal gets its unique colouring from small bubbles of quartz underneath its surface. It is considered a gentler, more "feminine" variety of the quartz family, at least when compared to the "masculine" clear quartz. This softer energy can be used to align and balance the chakras during meditative practice.

This stone is well known for its emotional healing properties and its ability to reduce stress. It is also prized for its capacity to boost memory and self-confidence, drawing in negative energies and radiating positivity.

CRYSTAL TIPS

Place this stone on the skin, either as jewellery or in your hand, to protect against overwhelming thoughts and feelings entering the mind.

Use this stone during meditation to help expand your practice. The crystal is thought to heighten intuition and facilitate deeper thinking by activating the crown chakra; this, in turn, allows for a deeper connection with the higher self.

Keep this stone close at hand, perhaps in your purse or somewhere in your living area, to help ease uncomfortable symptoms pertaining to the menstrual cycle.

Moonstone

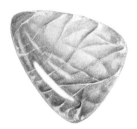

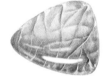

Origin: Brazil, India, Germany, Sri Lanka, Madagascar, Myanmar, Mexico, Tanzania and the US

Colour: Opalescent variants of blue, grey, white, pink or green

Birthstone for: June

Chakra zone: Heart, third eye and crown

Best for: Stability, divinity and sensuality

This mysterious and enchanting stone has been prized by many cultures throughout history for its moon-like sheen. It has a particularly feminine and sensual aura, channelling the soothing and peaceful energies of the moon; reminiscent of its ebbs and flows, moonstone calms and encourages, teaching the natural rhythms of life in accordance with the world around us. The clearer and more colourful the stone, the more healing its energies are thought to be.

CRYSTAL TIPS

Use this crystal in a place clear from clutter and distractions. Meditate on your intentions and your goals for the near future, and repeat this ritual every full moon in order to experience the full benefit of this stone.

Wear moonstone when you feel you need to be opened up to new love and sensitivity. As a stone of eroticism and fertility, it is advisable to wear it during intimate encounters to align with the natural lunar cycle.

Cleanse the stone gently and often, limiting its exposure to sunlight, and recharge it under the light of the full moon. By taking care of the stone, you will maximize its healing energies.

Obsidian

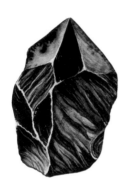

Origin: The US, Canada, Mexico, Guatemala, Argentina, Chile, Greece, Hungary, Italy, Iceland, Russia, New Zealand, Japan and Kenya

Colour: Black

Birthstone for: November

Chakra zone: Root

Best for: Self-reflection, growth and protection

Obsidian is a crystal best known for its stabilizing and grounding effects. Although it's linked with the concept of darkness, it is a powerful protective stone which allows self-reflection of the darker traits in your personality. Through this reflective process, obsidian shines a light on negativity and offers healing qualities. The crystal's powers of catharsis and deep soul-healing impel personal growth and resolution, and lend support during this process. It is highly protective, shielding from negativity in the environment, from others and from within the self.

CRYSTAL TIPS

Wear an obsidian arrow on a necklace to counter negativity toward you and to protect yourself against bullying. Alternatively, place small and pointed arrows of this stone in your workplace to ward off spiteful behaviour. In each case, this stone will offer a constant flow of tough and resilient energy.

Hold a stone in each hand when you feel as though you are torn between competing priorities in your life, in order to feel harmony restored to your root chakra – the centre which roots you to the earth.

Carry this stone with you while you are going through a healing process. It will offer the strength and patience needed to overcome challenges in your life.

Onyx

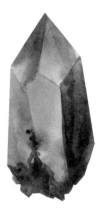

Origin: **Yemen, Central and South America, Australia, Canada, China, Czech Republic, Germany, India, Indonesia, Madagascar and the UK**

Colour: **Black**

Birthstone for: **July**

Chakra zone: **Root, solar plexus and third eye**

Best for: **Protection, calm and release**

Onyx is a protective stone which should be worn when facing adversities or uncertain situations, or to act as a defence against negative energies – internal or external. Historically, this stone has been used for its protective qualities and to impart courage to its wearer; Indians and Persians, in particular, used to believe that wearing an onyx protected them from the evil eye, while

Romans would wear this stone into battle for courage. Onyx is thought to bring increased vigour, strength, stamina and self-control. The stone alleviates worry, tension and fear, and eliminates confusion.

CRYSTAL TIPS

Wear onyx jewellery to bolster your confidence and encourage forward progress in your life. Alternatively, keep an onyx crystal with you throughout times of uncertainty or when you feel your emotional strength waver.

- -

Place an onyx stone in a glass of water and then drink the elixir to feel healing vibrations in your body – just remember to take out the stone before drinking. These vibrations will instil a sense of calm and provide a release from periods of anxiety.

- -

Hold an onyx crystal or figurine in your hand while you meditate and focus on it in your practice to clear your mind and facilitate a strong connection with spiritual guidance.

Opal

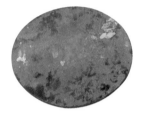

Origin: **Australia, Mexico, Brazil, Indonesia, Czech Republic, Ethiopia and the US**

Colour: **Iridescent in colours including yellow, orange, green, blue, red and purple**

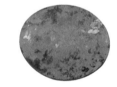

Birthstone for: **October**

Chakra zone: **Crown**

Best for: **Optimism, reflection and calm**

Derived from the Latin *opalus*, meaning "precious stone", the opal has traditionally been linked with good luck and hope. The stone amplifies our feelings and desires, and reflects them back to ourselves – much as the opal absorbs and reflects the light which surrounds it. The stone reminds us of the joy of our earthly existence and bolsters our zest for life. Opal crystals also soothe restless minds, and relieve anxiety and stress.

CRYSTAL TIPS

During meditation, hold a piece of opal in each hand to promote a calm and centred mind, and to help you to connect with the earth and its spirit. As common opals vibrate at a lower frequency, they are able to ground the emotional body to ease stress and bring tranquillity.

Wear this stone when you wish to arouse desire in yourself and those around you. As a highly seductive stone, opal will intensify your emotional state and help you to let go of your inhibitions.

Keep this stone nearby when you require emotional stability, as opal will support level-headedness and a mature attitude, reminding you to take responsibility for your emotional state.

Peridot

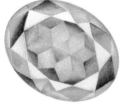

Origin: Australia, Brazil, China, Egypt, Kenya, Mexico, Myanmar, Norway, Pakistan and the US

Colour: Green

Birthstone for: August

Chakra zone: Heart

Best for: Happiness, prosperity and abundance

According to legend, the peridot was a favourite stone of Queen Cleopatra, who wore it both for its beauty and its powers of protection against evil spirits. Created from the intense inferno of volcanoes, peridot is believed to be a gift from Mother Nature and is widely considered to be a symbol of the planet's yearly renewal. The luminous and lush greens of the stone are reminiscent of nature and springtime, and they evoke feelings of joy and optimism in its wearer. The stone is known to bolster a sense of self-worth and motivation, as well as increasing prosperity.

CRYSTAL TIPS

Place peridot over your heart chakra to clear blockages from this region; you will be more open to relationships with others and more willing to make yourself emotionally vulnerable.

Wear a ring or bracelet with peridot stones on your dominant hand or wrist to harness the power of the stone on a daily basis. This will be particularly beneficial during challenging emotional periods, such as when you are changing jobs or going through conflict in your personal life; peridot offers an optimistic outlook and a balanced view of the world.

Take time to gaze at this stone and to admire its glimmering, forest-green beauty.

Pyrite

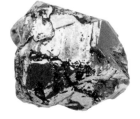

Origin: **Spain and the US**

Colour: **Gold**

Birthstone for: **July**

Chakra zone: **Solar plexus**

Best for: **Personal growth and confidence**

Treasured by a number of ancient civilizations, this shimmering, golden stone manifests passionate energy, and acts as a symbol of abundance and prosperity. The word pyrite comes from the Greek *pyr*, meaning "fire". Also known as "fool's gold" for its metallic and brass-yellow appearance, this stone has historically been used in ritual ceremonies and divination, as well as in ornamental objects.

Pyrite guards against negative behaviours and helps to deflect harm, as well as inspiring harmony and balance. The crystal stirs a sense of ambition, perseverance, self-worth and motivation.

CRYSTAL TIPS

Place a piece of this crystal in your workplace to bring prosperity and abundance to your working environment, and to attract wealth and success to your endeavours. The stone will bring fresh energy, and impart an immediate increase in vitality and self-confidence.

Wear jewellery made of pyrite, such as a necklace or brooch, to help improve circulatory and upper respiratory function.

Carry a pyrite worry stone in your purse or pocket when you feel that you are anxious or intimidated by a situation. The crystal will ease your apprehension and allow you to feel calm within yourself.

Rhodonite

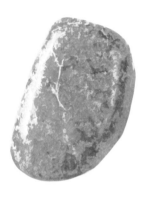

Origin: **Australia, Finland, Japan, Canada, Madagascar, Mexico, Russia, Sweden, South Africa, Tanzania and the US**

Colour: **Pink to red, with black speckling**

Birthstone for: **May**

Chakra zone: **Heart**

Best for: **Forgiveness, love and emotional healing**

Known as the "rescue stone", rhodonite is one of the most powerful heart chakra crystals in the gem world, working therapeutically to bolster compassion and forgiveness in times of heightened emotion. Acting almost as a lens through which to see your situation, this stone stimulates empathy in times of anger, distress and conflict. It is often used as a healing stone for relationships, encouraging clear communication and forming healthy, open unions. Rhodonite replaces anxiety, fear and anger with feelings of self-worth and emotional well-being, allowing you to experience true happiness.

CRYSTAL TIPS

Wear this stone as jewellery – in a long pendant or brooch, if possible – in order to best channel your heart chakra and to feel the maximum benefit from the crystal. By doing this, all the energies relating to this chakra, including love, peace and decision-making, will filter through the stone to the outside world.

Place a piece of this stone under your mattress to harness its protective power while you are sleeping, as it will help to ensure your safety and well-being during the night. It is also a good idea to keep this stone around in the bedroom, if you wish to channel its romantic and sensual energies with your partner.

Rose quartz

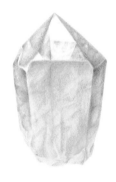

Origin: **Madagascar, India, Japan, Brazil, South Africa and the US**

Colour: **Pink**

Birthstone for: **January**

Chakra zone: **Heart**

Best for: **Matters of the heart and calming friction in relationships of all kinds**

Rose quartz has a gentle blush-pink colour and is known as the crystal for matters of the heart. It emits powerful, nurturing vibrations to your heart chakra, which can be used to boost self-love, emotional balance, friendship and romance. It helps to lower stress levels and dissipate feelings of resentment, upset and jealousy.

CRYSTAL TIPS

The rose quartz stone can be used as part of a daily morning meditation; try this simple exercise to promote instant calm. Think of a positive word to use as your mantra – it could be something like "peace", "happy" or "calm". Sit on the floor with your legs crossed loosely or stretched out – whichever is most comfortable. Hold your rose quartz stone in your dominant hand and rest your hands in your lap. Close your eyes and feel the soothing vibrations of the stone, as you take in deep breaths. Say your positive mantra each time you exhale. Do this for 5 minutes as a wonderful way to prepare yourself for the day ahead.

- -

Place small pieces of rose quartz throughout your home and workplace to help disperse negative energies, and promote feelings of joy and togetherness.

- -

Wear a rose quartz pendant to ease stress and encourage calm.

Ruby

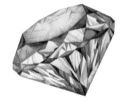

Origin: Thailand, Cambodia, Myanmar, India, Afghanistan, Australia, Namibia, Colombia, Japan, Scotland, Brazil and Pakistan

Colour: Red

Birthstone for: July

Chakra zone: Root and heart

Best for: Passion, protection and prosperity

Ruby is a stone that has been treasured and revered throughout history for its captivating colour and powerful aura. This crystal has always stood as a talisman of passion and prosperity, symbolizing the glowing hues of the sun and the colour of blood. Today, the stone is valued for its ability to offer vitality to those who wear it, as it stimulates the circulation and amplifies the energies within us. Ruby is also a popular stone for signifying love – whether to kindle a new romance or to lose yourself in the throes of passion, it is a powerful amplifier.

CRYSTAL TIPS

Wear this stone when you feel low or depleted to help enhance your motivation and encourage you to set practical goals. Given its strong association with romance and desire, this stone also gives a powerful boost to your sexual energy, encouraging vitality and sensuality in those around it.

Keep this stone nearby when tackling difficult or emotionally charged situations to provide you with feelings of strength and resolve. Ruby crystals bring out your most courageous and positive states of mind, drawing out the protective aspects of your character and helping you to stand up for what you believe in.

Rutilated quartz

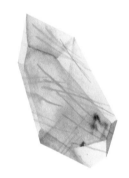

Origin: Australia, Brazil, Kazakhstan, Madagascar, Norway, Pakistan and the US

Colour: Yellow and brown

Birthstone for: April

Chakra zone: Third eye

Best for: Clarity, energy and strength

This quartz is often colourless, and characterized by the presence of "needles" or strands of rutile within its structure. Also called Venus's hair stone because of these golden strands, the ancients were just as drawn to its glistening lustre as we are today. While quartz promotes positive energy, rutile strongly improves awareness of the world, thus forming a truly potent psychic stone. This stone delivers powerful cleansing and purifying effects.

CRYSTAL TIPS

Keep this crystal nearby while you are meditating to help develop psychic gifts. As this quartz energizes the higher mind, it may assist you in receiving spiritual knowledge and guidance, and help you to gain concentration and mental clarity. It is useful to keep a journal close by to write down any thoughts that come to mind after meditating with the stone, as you will be able to face the truth of your emotions and the negative thoughts holding you back.

Wear this stone in jewellery to utilize its powers of manifestation. Given its strong vibrations, it is open to being programmed with your intentions, which may assist you to move your life forward quickly in your desired direction.

Selenite

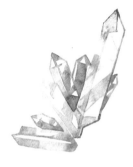

Origin: **Mexico, Australia, Greece, Madagascar and the US**

Colour: **White, translucent**

Birthstone for: **September**

Chakra zone: **Crown**

Best for: **Cleansing, clarity and light**

The name of this crystal derives from the ancient Greek word for "moon" *(selene),* which is apt for its milky-white hue. Both in look and energy, this stone is one of the purest in the crystal world, and as such is very effective in absorbing negative energies from around it. It is also popularly used for purifying and recharging other crystals. Its high vibrational energy makes it an effective stone for enhancing self-awareness. For this reason, the stone is also excellent when used in meditation, as it helps to provide insights and an awareness of your spiritual journey.

CRYSTAL TIPS

Use this crystal to cleanse your other stones whenever you feel as if their energy is dull or perhaps less vibrant than it used to be. Lay them on top of a large selenite block to recharge overnight.

Run selenite crystals up and down your body while visualizing them taking away your negativity, worries and stresses from the day, and to feel lighter and clear-headed.

Place selenite crystals throughout your house – particularly in places where you require clear and pure energy – to shift the energies from negative to positive.

Smoky quartz

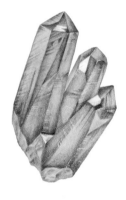

Origin: Brazil, Madagascar, Mozambique, Australia, Switzerland, Scotland and the US

Colour: Greyish-brown to black

Birthstone for: June

Chakra zone: Root

Best for: Healing, grounding and letting go

While seemingly not as popular as some other quartz crystals, namely the clear and rose varieties, this stone offers a great number of benefits. With a strong connection to the root chakra, it is particularly effective as an anchoring stone to the earth, helping to expand awareness of the surrounding world and improving survival instincts. This stone is also ideal for those carrying emotional baggage, as smoky quartz helps to ease negativity and conflict.

CRYSTAL TIPS

Wear smoky quartz as a necklace to stimulate and balance your chakras, and to help you to feel grounded. This stone is grounding in a uniquely uplifting way, providing a subtler energy than other balancing gemstones.

Meditate while holding a piece of smoky quartz in each hand to receive deep insight and guidance during your practice.

Keep this stone nearby to harness its protective qualities and to allow it to draw out negative energies from the space you are in.

Sunstone

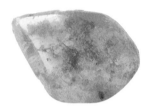

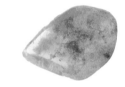

Origin: Australia, Canada, China, Congo, India, Mexico, Norway, Russia, Sri Lanka, Tanzania and the US

Colour: Yellow, red and orange hues

Birthstone for: August

Chakra zone: Sacral

Best for: Healing, sensuality and happiness

Known as a joyful stone, this crystal inspires self-care and the inclination to help others. Sunstone restores enjoyment of life, while also providing a sense of abundance. With its strong solar energy, it is a powerful stone for bringing joy, warmth and strength, as well as helping to reduce stress and negative thought patterns, and aiding digestive issues.

CRYSTAL TIPS

Wear jewellery made with sunstone to assist with breaking away from toxic relationships and to sever the bonds that are holding you back in life. The energy of this stone may also enhance your intuition, thus helping you to avoid forming similar toxic bonds in future.

- -

Keep this stone around you in your work environment to help filter out dishonesty in your colleagues and clients.

- -

Look upon this stone each day when you wake up, and allow it to fill your soul with energy and joy. By bolstering your self-worth and confidence, sunstone is your natural supplement for life.

Tiger's eye

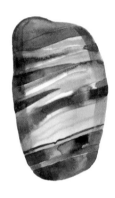

Origin: South Africa, Thailand, Canada, Western Australia, Spain, Brazil, China, Myanmar, India and the US

Colour: Yellow and brown

Birthstone for: August

Chakra zone: Root, sacral and solar plexus

Best for: Good fortune, prosperity and inspiration

Resembling the eye of a tiger, this crystal contains the energy of both the earth and the sun. Tiger's eye is known for bringing luck and prosperity, acting as an "all-seeing eye", which is thought to imbue the wearer with self-confidence and allow them to deflect the malice of others around them. This stone also offers power and emotional stability when working through lifestyle changes, as well as reducing the anxiety that surrounds them. Tiger's eye is also thought to stimulate creativity in artists and to encourage "thinking outside the box".

CRYSTAL TIPS

Wear this stone as jewellery to keep the crystal close to your chakras – for instance in a ring, bracelet or as a pendant. The vibrations will stimulate passion, energy and good fortune, as well as relieving emotional stress.
Keep this stone around at times when you feel like you are losing control in your life, and need to restore balance and harmony. It will help to stabilize your physical and emotional well-being.

Pair this stone with your favourite quartz crystal to magnify its effect on you.

Tourmaline

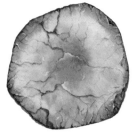

Origin: Brazil, Tanzania, Nigeria, Kenya, Madagascar, Mozambique, Namibia, Afghanistan, Pakistan, Sri Lanka and Malawi

Colour: A variety, but mainly black, brown, blue, yellow, green and pink

Birthstone for: October

Chakra zone: Root

Best for: Cleansing, grounding and protection

Popularly seen as a protective stone, tourmaline has long been used as a talisman, offering safety, cleansing and grounding to those who possess it. Tourmaline emits a supportive energy, which aligns the energy centres of the body and channels healing, both physically and mentally. The stone also offers a sense of power and self-confidence, so is often carried in difficult circumstances and challenging situations. One of the most powerful of these tourmaline stones is the black variety, which offers all of the above benefits.

CRYSTAL TIPS

Hold a piece of tourmaline in your hand for a few minutes when you feel that you need to boost your concentration and dispel distractions around you.

Place a tourmaline stone in your home or workplace to soothe you and guard against stressors. It is also useful for protecting you against toxic friends, who might wish to drain your energy and offer little in return.

Keep a tourmaline stone near you during meditation to help cleanse your mind of negative thoughts, anxieties and feelings of anger. As this stone is closely linked with the root chakra, it is also useful as a grounding tool, keeping you closely tied to the physical plane.

Turquoise

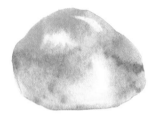

Origin: Iran, Afghanistan, China, Australia, Chile, Mexico and the US

Colour: Blue-green

Birthstone for: December

Chakra zone: All chakras

Best for: Health, wisdom and protection

This gem has been used for making jewellery, statues, amulets and even architecture since before 5000 BC. Turquoise is associated with personal protection and, due to its dazzling colour, has historically been seen as a stone of good fortune.

As well as bringing a pop of vibrancy, this stone lifts the spirits and promotes well-being by energizing all chakra centres.

CRYSTAL TIPS

Wear turquoise in jewellery or keep it close to the body to support inner peace and harmony, as well as easing uncertainty and anxieties in your life. Simply holding the stone for a few seconds can calm the mind and help to realign your focus and intentions. This stone is also particularly effective when worn in a necklace, due to the proximity it then has to the heart; keeping it close to your body in this way boosts its healing effects and allows it to act as a life-affirming force.

Place this stone over your third eye chakra during meditation to aid clairvoyant abilities. This practice will also help you to go deeper in to your meditation and communicate with your inner truth.

Unakite

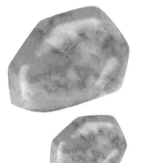

Origin: South Africa, Sierra Leone, Brazil, China and the US

Colour: Green and pink

Birthstone for: Associated with springtime

Chakra zone: Third eye

Best for: Positivity, awareness and release

Named after the Unaka Mountains of North Carolina, where it was first discovered, unakite is considered to be a stone that deepens meditative practice by awakening you to the present moment. This stone helps to release the pain and regret of the past, and awakens a new, spiritual life, with an awareness of the brevity of time.

Unakite brings together the nurturing spirit of green with the soft, caring aspect of pink to form one of nature's most healing crystals. The stone resonates with the frequency of love, compassion and kindness.

CRYSTAL TIPS

Keep a piece of unakite near to you while you are engaging in hobbies, such as gardening, cooking or going to the gym, in order to maximize the enjoyment in what you are doing. The stone will also inspire you to work hard and improve yourself on the path toward achieving measurable success.

Wear this stone as a gentle reminder of time, which is constantly flowing and impossible to cling on to. Keeping this around you will incentivize you to seize the day and to make the most of every moment.

Yellow fluorite

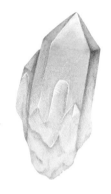

Origin: **Argentina, the UK, Germany, India, Morocco, Namibia, Spain and the US**

Colour: **Yellow**

Birthstone for: **July**

Chakra zone: **Solar plexus and third eye**

Best for: **Happiness, creativity and focus**

Soft, luminous and glassy, yellow fluorite often occurs in extraordinary tightly stacked cubes. This stone carries a calm and stable frequency which brings order to chaos, and fosters deep thought and concentration. Yellow fluorite stirs creativity and clears mental confusion, as well as easing anxiety. Fluorite (see page 48) is particularly effective as a "focus stone", used for maintaining discipline in daily life and exercise routines, engendering strength and endurance.

CRYSTAL TIPS

Hold a piece of yellow fluorite in your hands as you meditate or relax to feel a sense of calm and serenity within you. This is also an effective way to strengthen your connection to the earth.

- -

Rotate a yellow fluorite tumbled stone clockwise around your body as an aura cleanser. You can also use it to stimulate your third eye chakra, and to boost psychic communication and promote spiritual balance.

- -

Simply look at this stone and appreciate its radiant hue to benefit from its healing and calming energies, and to stimulate a brighter and more positive outlook on life. Use it in an elixir or wear it on the body to keep daydreaming to a minimum in workplace environments or situations requiring focus.

Zircon

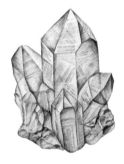

Origin: Norway, Pakistan, Cambodia, Myanmar, Thailand, Sri Lanka, Australia, France, Vietnam, Tanzania, Russia, Madagascar, Canada and the US

Colour: Reddish-brown, yellow, green, blue, grey and clear

Birthstone for: December

Chakra zone: All chakras

Best for: Joy, protection and vitality

Often confused with cubic zirconia, zircon is its own crystal and has been prized for centuries as a stone of protection. Though many stones are heat treated to increase their colour intensity, natural hues vary from deep red to grey and from blue to golden yellow. These crystals embody a strong healing energy and have an effective spiritual grounding vibration. Zircon helps to balance virtuous aspects within you and has a strong effect on all of your chakras.

CRYSTAL TIPS

Hold a stone in each hand during meditation to keep you from feeling unbalanced or spaced-out. Zircon is known for having a strong grounding force, so will help to restore harmony in your physical body, as well as providing emotional and spiritual stability.

Wear this stone next to your skin, rather than inside a pocket or in a bag, in your daily life to fortify your positivity and protect against harmful negative forces around you.

Place this stone over your chakras to stimulate sluggish energies to move down toward the earth. This may help to relieve feelings of anxiety, and cleanse your body and mind from the stressors coming from the world around you.

EVERY PARTICULAR IN NATURE, A LEAF, A DROP, A CRYSTAL, A MOMENT OF TIME IS RELATED TO THE WHOLE, AND PARTAKES OF THE PERFECTION OF THE WHOLE.

RALPH WALDO EMERSON

SELF-CARE
with Crystals

In this section we explore simple self-care procedures and rituals that you can incorporate into everyday life to help you get the most from your crystals.

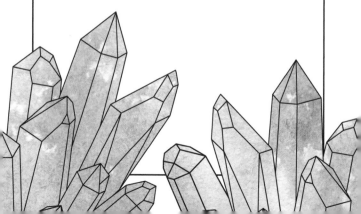

CREATE A SACRED SPACE IN YOUR HOUSE WITH CRYSTALS

Crystals can transform the energy of a space and create a calming atmosphere for meditations and relaxation. A sacred space in the home is important to help nurture creativity, and for regular moments of self-care and reflection. Here are a few simple steps to creating your own sanctuary with crystals.

Begin by choosing a place away from the hustle and bustle of home life. It could be an area of your living room or bedroom, or a sheltered place in the garden – somewhere you won't be disturbed and can feel at ease. Make sure there is a comfortable place to sit.

Clear the space of "dead energy" by allowing air to flow through (if it's indoors), and clearing away dust, dirt and cobwebs. Then declutter the area so there are only a few valued items close by. Calming scented candles are a nice option.

Next, add some crystals that will calm the energies in the space – amethyst or different types of quartz, such as rose and clear, work particularly well, as they are good for cleansing, healing and harmony.

Place the crystals where they will catch and reflect natural light, and give each one sufficient space.

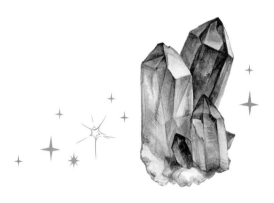

CRYSTALS ARE LIVING BEINGS AT THE BEGINNING OF CREATION.

NIKOLA TESLA

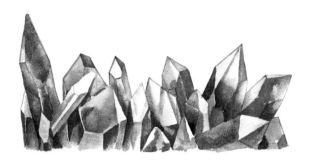

TRY A CRYSTAL MEDITATION

If you are experiencing a particular imbalance or problem, look up the relevant crystal/chakra to focus on (or use one for each chakra and perform a general balancing meditation). Lie down comfortably and place your crystal over or next to the corresponding chakra. Take some slow breaths and then visualize coloured healing energy emanating from the crystal and flowing through your body. (Work from the root chakra up, if you are balancing all the chakras.)

LOVE SPELL

Crystals are a popular resource when casting spells for white witchcraft – be reassured that this is about making magic with only good intentions. Try this simple love ritual, which is designed to give your romantic life a boost.

You will need
- Two pieces of rose quartz
- Two pink candles
- A photo of you and your partner

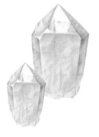

Find a quiet place in your home where you won't be disturbed. Light the candles, and think about your partner and what you love about them. Allow the candles to burn down and place the rose quartz stones under your bed. Practise this spell on a new, waxing or full moon on any given day.

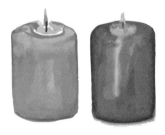

AN ABUNDANCE RITUAL

Crystals serve to amplify your positive intentions – if you are in need of a boost to your financial wealth, try this simple ritual.

You will need
- A small piece of pyrite
- Something that represents your business or a work-related goal, such as a contract, a job advert or a business card
- Your workspace

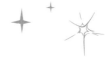

Begin by carefully selecting your stone. Feel which one resonates with you, before cleansing it in either running water or sunlight (see page 22). Take the pyrite to your workspace and, while you gently hold it in your hand, consider the goal that you are trying to reach and invite the abundant energy within the pyrite to assist with your endeavour. Focus on your goal for a few minutes, without distraction, and then place the pyrite on the item that you have chosen to represent what you would like to achieve. Keep the crystal visible on your desk or in the room where you work – or your car, if you don't have a sedentary job – so that the energy from the pyrite resonates throughout the space.

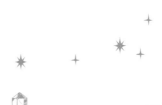

MAKE A CRYSTAL WISH BAG

This is a lovely intuitive and creative form of spell-casting, and it's also one of the nicest ways to perform a spell for another person. It takes time but the results – as long as the intentions are good – are worth it.

You will need
- A small drawstring bag (this can be handmade or shop-bought)
- A crystal of your choosing
- A charm that resonates with you or your friend (optional)
- A piece of paper and a pen
- A candle

Wish bags traditionally contain one or more objects that can then be carried discreetly in a pocket or handbag. Elements that can be used include crystals or semi-precious stones and small items significant to a spell, such as a small carved object, earth, seeds or pips – the options are infinite. The wish bags are often made from red felt, but any fabric can be used and it's up to you how elaborate you make it; the intention should be written clearly on a sheet of white paper, which is folded and placed inside the bag. Choose stones that contain the properties that you or your friend require assistance with, such as tiger's eye for a confidence boost before a job interview or important event, or smoky quartz to heal a rift in a relationship or ease a separation.

To charge your wish bag with magical energy, place it next to a candle. Light the candle and focus your energy on visualizing the outcome of the spell, or imagine the obstacles falling away in order for you to reach your goal. These spells can be performed over several days, until the candle has burned down; then you can carry your wish bag around with you until the spell has worked. Alternatively, if it is for a friend in need, give them the wish bag and a candle. Instruct them to light the candle, when they have a quiet moment, and focus on their wish while holding the bag. The candle can be lit over several days until it has burned down. Encourage your friend to keep the wish bag with them: on their desk or bedside table, or in a pocket or handbag.

Ideas for charms to place in your wish bag

Acorn: luck, prosperity and sexual potency

Clover: life, luck and abundance

Horn: repels the evil eye; it is a symbol of nature, fertility and sexuality

Horseshoe: luck

Key: power and luck, especially if it is found and the finder does not know which lock it opens; a symbol of access to hidden things

Lightning-struck wood: protection against all harm

Pine cone: luck, favourable influences and protection from harm; it also repels bad influences

Religious symbol: symbols of various religions are considered to be protective

Salt: purification; it repels evil

Silver: protection and wealth

CRYSTALS AMPLIFY THE CONSCIOUSNESS.

SHIRLEY MACLAINE

BIRTHSTONES BY MONTH

The tradition of birthstones dates back thousands of years, to the Book of Exodus. In the 1st century BC, Jewish historian Josephus believed there was a connection between the twelve stones in Aaron's breastplate, the twelve months of the year and the twelve signs of the zodiac. Since then, many scholars have identified the stones which best align with each month, ascribing zodiacal traits to each gem. Wearing your birthstone is thought to offer health, happiness and prosperity, all year round, alongside the more specific benefits the stone can offer you.

January
Garnet
Jet
Milky quartz
Rose quartz

February
Amethyst
Hematite
(and April)

March
Aquamarine
Jade
Jasper

April
Clear quartz
Diamond
Hematite
Rutilated quartz

May
Amber
Beryl
Rhodonite

June
Agate
Blue lace agate
Moonstone
Smoky quartz

July
Chrysoprase
Onyx
Pyrite
Ruby
Yellow fluorite

August
Carnelian
Labradorite
Peridot
Sunstone
Tiger's eye

September
Aventurine
Lapis lazuli
Selenite

October
Opal
Tourmaline

November
Citrine
Obsidian

December
Turquoise
Zircon

CONCLUSION

This book has introduced you to the many wonderful holistic properties of crystals. Crystals vary incredibly in colour, opalescence and texture – each one is unique and has its own magic – and for this reason it can take a lifetime to discover the benefits of each one. Enjoy the journey as you discover the crystals pertinent to you and your needs.

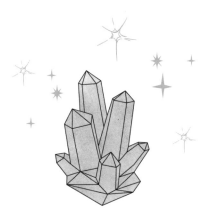

FURTHER READING

CRYSTAL HEALING

Hall, Judy *101 Power Crystals* (2001, Fair Winds Press)

Mercier, Patricia *The Chakra Bible* (2009, Godsfield Press)

Permutt, Philip *Crystal Tips and Cures* (2015, CICO Books)

Saradananda, Swami *Chakra Meditation* (2011, Watkins Publishing)

CRYSTALS AND WHITE WITCHCRAFT

Basile, Lisa Marie and Sollee, Kristen J. *Light Magic for Dark Times* (2018, Fair Winds Press)

Carvel, Astrid *The Little Book of Spells* (2019, Summersdale)

Carvel, Astrid *The Little Book of Witchcraft* (2017, Summersdale)

Grant, Ember *The Book of Crystal Spells* (2013, Llewellyn Publications)

CRYSTALS INDEX

If you're interested in finding out more about our books, find us on Facebook at **Summersdale Publishers** and follow us on Twitter at **@Summersdale**.

WWW.SUMMERSDALE.COM

Image credits